Beginner-Friendly Jelqing Exercises

Beginner-friendly Jelqing Exercises and Effective Techniques For Mastering Male Enhancement Safely and Effectively.

Title:
Beginner-Friendly Jelqing Exercises

Subtitle

Beginner-friendly Jelqing Exercises and Effective Techniques For Mastering Male Enhancement Safely and Effectively.

Copyright © 2024 by (Josue Collins)

Printed in the United States of America.

ISBN: 9798876887481

TABLE OF CONTENT

INTRODUCTION

This is not just about pursuing physical improvement; it is a gateway to adopting a holistic approach to male sexual health. If you go on the journey of studying Jelq exercises and implementing them into your life, you are not simply seeking physical enhancement. In this extensive introduction, we will delve into the core aspects that form the foundation of our investigation. These core aspects include defining Jelqing, examining its historical roots, and elaborating on the myriad of benefits that it can bring to the lives of men who are looking to improve their sexual wellness.

What is Jelqing?

One of the most important aspects of this book is the technique that is referred to as Jelqing. Although many people may not be familiar with this phrase, it strikes a chord with individuals who are looking for natural ways to improve their sexual functioning. To increase the amount of blood that flows to the penis, jelqing is a manual exercise that has its origins in ancient traditions and has been improved over time. This technique entails making controlled and rhythmic strokes along the length of the penis while it is in a semi-erect position.

When jelqing is performed, mild pressure is regularly given to the penis. This motion is sometimes referred to as a "milking" motion. The approach does not stress acts that are quick and aggressive; rather, it emphasizes a process that is steady and deliberate. To get the desired results, the objective is to stimulate the circulation of blood into the erectile tissues, which may result in enhancements to the penile girth and general sexual performance.

Jelqing is firmly embedded in cultural and historical settings, and its origins can be traced back to a variety of civilizations all over the world. While the notion may appear to be original to some people, it is crucial to acknowledge that Jelqing has been around for a very long time.

Historical Overview

To get a complete understanding of the significance of Jelqing, one must travel back into the annals of history. In those times, ancient societies understood the relevance of sexual health and looked for natural ways to improve virility.

Jelqing is a religious practice that has its roots in the traditions of ancient Arabic culture, notably in the context of Islamic sexual health. Historical literature, such as the "Kama Sutra" from ancient India, also refers to manual exercises that are intended to increase the sexual prowess of men. In many cases, these activities were linked with more general ideas concerning the state of one's bodily health and spiritual equilibrium.

In a similar vein, in traditional Chinese medicine, where the interconnection of the body's energy pathways is of the utmost importance, it was believed that exercises that were similar to Jelqing would increase not just sexual vitality but also general vitality.

As we go deeper into the historical origins of Jelqing, it becomes abundantly clear that this practice is not a fad but rather a time-honored custom that has persisted throughout the millennia. Even though the methods and cultural circumstances may differ, the fundamental premise of improving male sexual

health continues to be a consistent theme.

Benefits of Jelq Exercise

Beyond the historical fabric, Jelqing's appeal is derived from the multitude of advantages it may present to people who are dedicated to practicing it. Let's examine the many benefits of jelqing, which are causing men to look for natural ways to improve their sex to become more interested in learning more about it.

- Enhanced Blood Flow: The idea behind Jelqing is to improve blood flow to the penis. People who perform this exercise want to activate the erectile tissues and blood vessels, which may result in increased blood flow. Improved circulation may benefit general penile health in addition to supporting erectile performance.

- Potential Girth Enhancement: Promoting penile girth is one of Jelqing's main goals. By means of regular, regulated exercise, people want to promote the growth of the erectile tissues, which will lead to a bigger penis. Some practitioners report good increases in penile girth over time, while individual results may vary.

- Enhanced Erectile Function: It is commonly known that blood flow and erectile function are related. Improvements in erectile function may be experienced by persons who incorporate Jelqing into their regimen. This may be especially important for people who have mild to moderate erectile dysfunction.

- Increased Sexual Confidence: Jelqing's all-encompassing method, which addresses the mental and physical facets of sexual health, may help boost one's self-assurance in one's sexual abilities. People's confidence naturally rises when they observe favorable changes in their physique and sexual performance.

- Non-Invasive and Natural: Jelqing is a unique method of male enhancement that is both non-invasive and natural. Jelqing doesn't require any extra equipment or drugs, in contrast to pharmacological or surgical methods. Those looking for options with fewer possible adverse effects will find this appealing.

- Cultural and Historical Connection: Jelqing's allure for certain people extends beyond its health benefits. The understanding that this technique has its origins in antiquated customs and has been handed down through the ages gives the process of self-improvement a cultural and historical context.

UNDERSTANDING MALE ANATOMY

When beginning the path of Jelq exercises, it is necessary to have a full awareness of male anatomy. By looking into the deep aspects of the male reproductive system, particularly the penis, we can gain an understanding of the physiological basis upon which Jelqing functions. In the course of this investigation, we will examine the shape of the penis, uncover the intricate systems that are responsible for blood flow and erections, and emphasize the significant role that circulation plays in ensuring that sexual health is maintained at its highest possible level.

The Structure of the Penis

It is the outstanding organ that is responsible for reproduction and sexual function and is located at the center of the male anatomy. This organ is the penis. Having a fundamental understanding of its anatomy is essential to appreciate how Jelqing, a technique that is founded in increasing blood flow to this organ, may alter the form and function of this organ.

- Three cylindrical columns of erectile tissue make up the penis: the corpora cavernosa, which are two bigger columns, and the corpus spongiosum, which is a smaller column. The corpus spongiosum encircles the urethra beneath the corpora cavernosa, which runs along the top side of the penis.

Erection maintenance and achievement depend on these structures.

- Glans and Urethra: The urethra, a duct that transports semen and urine, leaves the body at the rounded tip of the organ, the glans penis, after passing through the corpus spongiosum. The glans is a very delicate region that is essential to enjoying sex.

- Ligaments and Fascia: A variety of ligaments and fascia include connective tissues, which provide the penis its structural support. These components support the organ's general flexibility and form.

- Blood Vessels: An abundance of arteries and veins provide the penis with blood. The erectile tissues get oxygenated blood from arteries, and deoxygenated blood is returned to them through veins. The complex system of blood vessels plays a key role in the processes behind erection and flaccidity.

It is necessary to have an understanding of the micro and macroscopic characteristics of the penis to have a better understanding of how Jelqing affects these structures, which might potentially result in changes in girth and as well as general sexual function.

Blood Flow and Erection Mechanism

Erections are the result of a complex interaction between the neurological system, the vascular system, and the hormonal system. This interaction is called the "physiological foundations." It is vital to understand the complex systems that regulate blood flow and erections to have a complete understanding of the influence that Jelqing has on male sexual performance.

- Neurological Signals: A series of signals in the nervous system are set off by sexual excitement. These impulses, which are frequently brought on by sensory inputs, pass via the spinal cord and arrive in the genital region. There, they release neurotransmitters that cause the smooth muscle cells in the erectile tissues to relax.

- Arterial Dilation and Enhanced Blood Flow: When smooth muscles relax, the arteries dilate and more blood may enter the corpora cavernosa. The essential process underlying the outward display of an erection is the blood engorgement of these erectile chambers.

- Venous Compression: At the same time, the veins that carry blood out of the penis are compressed. By preventing blood from leaving the erectile tissues and keeping the penis tight during an erection, this compression keeps the erectile tissues under pressure.

- Function of Nitric Oxide: An essential signaling molecule, nitric oxide is essential to this process. By promoting smooth muscle relaxation, it helps to dilate blood vessels and improve blood flow. Numerous factors, such as cardiovascular health and physical activity level, affect nitric oxide production.

The possible impact of Jelqing can be better understood by first gaining an understanding of the complexities of blood flow and the process that causes an erection. Individuals who participate in Jelqing have the goal of optimizing the natural processes that lead to erectile function. This is accomplished by increasing increased blood flow to the penis to do regulated workouts.

Importance of Circulation for Sexual Health

The general idea behind Jelqing is to improve blood circulation to the penis, which is the primary focus of the practice. To fully appreciate the relevance of this emphasis, it is necessary to have a comprehensive understanding of the implications that circulation has for sexual health in general.

- Delivery of Nutrients and Oxygen: Healthy circulation is necessary to supply the penis's cells and tissues with needed nutrients and oxygen. The health of tissues as a whole and cellular metabolism depend on adequate oxygenation.

- Waste Removal: The elimination of waste items and metabolic wastes from the erectile tissues is made easier by efficient circulation. This procedure helps to keep the cellular environment in a healthy state.

- Temperature Regulation: The vaginal area's temperature is influenced by healthy blood circulation. Sperm function and general reproductive health depend on maintaining an ideal temperature.

- Endocrine System Interaction: Hormones and signaling molecules involved in sexual function are transported by the circulation. The regulation of several physiological processes depends on the interaction between the circulatory and endocrine systems.

- Preventing Erectile Dysfunction: One major cause of erectile dysfunction is impaired circulation. By putting cardiovascular health first and increasing blood flow with activities like Jelqing, people may be able to reduce their chance of experiencing erectile dysfunction.

Circulation is essential for sexual function, but its significance goes beyond that as it is fundamental to general health and well-being. Adopting circulation-boosting techniques like Jelqing is consistent with a holistic perspective on sexual well-being that acknowledges the interdependence of physiological systems.

GETTING STARTED WITH JELQING

When beginning the trip to Jelqing, it is necessary to approach it with careful consideration and knowledge. For those who are entering the world of Jelqing exercises for the very first time, this section is intended to serve as a guide. We provide the framework for a happy and productive experience with Jelqing by discussing safety considerations, creating reasonable expectations, and refuting common myths and misconceptions about the activity.

Safety Precautions

Prioritizing safety is necessary before beginning any Jelqing workouts. They are essential. Jelqing is usually regarded to be a safe technique when it is performed correctly; nevertheless, if it is not executed correctly or if it is performed with excessive enthusiasm, it might result in undesirable consequences. Important safety precautions to take into consideration are as follows:

- Talk with a Healthcare Expert: It's a good idea to speak with a healthcare professional before beginning any new workout program, particularly one that involves the genital area. For those who have pre-existing medical disorders or are concerned about their sexual health, this is especially crucial.

- Warm-Up Exercises: As with any physical exercise, it is important to warm up before beginning a Jelqing session. Mild warm-up techniques, such as gentle stretching and massage, assist in readying the penile tissues and lower the chance of harm.

- Gradual Progression and Moderation: Adopt a moderate and methodical approach while dealing with Jelqing. Do not overdo it, especially in the beginning. As your body adjusts, progressively boost the intensity and length of your Jelqing sessions. The right lubrication is crucial for jelqing because it minimizes friction and the chance of chafing or inflammation. Generally speaking, silicone- or water-based lubricants are advised.

- Technique Consistency: Maintaining consistency in technique is essential for both efficacy and safety. As stated in reliable manuals or educational resources, make sure you are using the correct Jelqing procedures. Steer clear of untested approaches while experimenting.

- Pay attention to your body: During and after Jelqing sessions, pay special attention to how your body reacts. If you feel any pain, discomfort, or strange feelings, stop doing the exercise. To avoid injuries, you must learn to listen to your body.

- Respect Individual Boundaries: Individual differences exist, and outcomes might differ. Be mindful of your own physiological and physical boundaries. Jelqing is not a foolproof technique for significant size increases, and pressing too hard might have unfavorable results.

- Cleanliness Procedures: Observe proper hygiene both before and following Jelqing. To avoid infection, make sure your hands and any tools you use are clean and thoroughly clean the genital region.

People may lay the groundwork for a secure and enjoyable Jelqing experience by following these safety guidelines. It is therefore imperative that we set reasonable expectations for the results of Jelqing as we go.

Setting Realistic Expectations

The possibility of achieving favorable changes in penile size and sexual function is frequently the driving force behind the popularity of Jelqing. However, to avoid disappointment and frustration, it is of the utmost importance to set reasonable expectations. Listed below are some important factors to take into account while setting reasonable expectations:

1. Individual Variability: People differ greatly in how they react to Jelqing. Results can be influenced by variables including heredity, general health, and exercise regimen adherence. Understand that different people will have different experiences.

2. Gradual Progression: Jelqing takes constant work over time; it's not a fast remedy. Anticipating abrupt and significant alterations might result in disillusionment. Instead, concentrate on small steps forward and advancements.

3. Length vs. Girth: Jelqing is more frequently linked to possible girth increase than length. Handling expectations is made easier by being aware of this difference. While some people may not notice significant changes in size, others may detect notable variations in girth.

4. General Sexual Health: Although increasing one's size is a typical objective, it's important to understand that Jelqing also benefits general sexual health. Better erection function enhanced blood flow and heightened sexual confidence are all worthwhile results that might not be quantified by size changes alone.

5. Combination with Other Practices: Take into account that Jelqing may provide greater all-encompassing advantages if it is included in a more comprehensive strategy for sexual well-being. Holistic well-being can be enhanced by incorporating Jelqing with other physical activities, a nutritious diet, and constructive sexual behavior.

6. Stressing Self-Discovery: Motivate people to see the Jelqing path as a process of self-care and self-discovery. Emphasize the possibilities for greater body awareness, sexual confidence, and a closer bond with one's own body rather than focusing just on physical improvements.

Individuals can approach Jelqing with a positive perspective so that they can acknowledge the diverse character of the practice. This is accomplished by cultivating reasonable expectations. Now, let's talk about some of the most widespread misunderstandings and fallacies that are related to jelqing.

Common Myths and Misconceptions

Jelqing, like many other procedures connected to sexual health, has amassed its fair share of myths and misconceptions over the years. These misunderstandings need to be dispelled for folks to be able to make educated judgments regarding whether or not to incorporate Jelqing into their daily routines. First, let's correct some common misconceptions:

Myth 1: Jelqing Promises a Size Gain

The reality is that jelqing is not a strategy that can completely ensure a large rise in size. A number of factors, including heredity, consistency in practice, and general health, all have a part in the outcomes that are experienced by different individuals. The reality is that jelqing is not a strategy that can completely ensure a large rise in size. A number of factors, including heredity, consistency in practice, and general health, all have a part in the outcomes that are experienced by different individuals.

Myth 2: Jelqing Causes Erectile Dysfunction

Jelqing is not known to cause erectile dysfunction when it is used appropriately, according to the reality sheet. It may contribute positively to sexual health since it will increase blood flow and improve erectile function.

Nevertheless, undesirable consequences may be brought about by the use of inappropriate procedures or excessive force.

Myth 3: Jelqing is a Rapid Solution

The reality is that jelqing is a procedure that takes time and requires consistency as well as patience. If you anticipate quick results, you can end yourself feeling frustrated. If you want to reap possible benefits, you need to practice consistently over a long period.

Myth 4: One Size Fits All Technique

The Jelqing technique may need to be modified to accommodate the tastes and reactions of each individual. There is no universally applicable strategy, and it may be necessary for individuals to experiment to determine what works best for them.

Myth 5: Jelqing Is Only About Size Enhancement

Although increasing one's size is a typical objective, Jelqing also makes a contribution to one's entire sexual health at the same time. A significant number of benefits, including enhanced blood flow, enhanced erection quality, and enhanced sexual confidence, are key components of the technique.

Myth 6: Jelqing Is a Substitute for Professional Advice

The reality is that jelqing should not be considered a replacement for the advice of a qualified medical practitioner. Before beginning Jelqing or any other new workout routine, those who have the presence of preexisting medical issues or who have concerns regarding their sexual health should seek the advice of a healthcare practitioner.

Individuals can approach Jelqing with a more comprehensive grasp of its potential advantages and limits if these beliefs are dispelled. To achieve sexual well-being, it is vital to approach the practice with an open mind, recognizing that the road toward sexual

wellness is varied and unique to each individual.

BASIC JELQING TECHNIQUES

To achieve mastery in the art of Jelqing, one must first comprehend and then put into practice a certain set of fundamental practices. We will cover warm-up exercises to prepare the penile tissues, provide a step-by-step guide to the Jelqing process, and emphasize the importance of finding one's comfort zone while performing these exercises. All of these topics will be covered in this comprehensive guide, which will cover the key aspects of basic Jelqing techniques.

Warm-up Exercises

Warming up before indulging in Jelqing is vital, just as it is before engaging in any other form of physical exercise, to prepare the tissues and reduce the likelihood of damage. Increasing the amount of blood that flows to the genital region with the use of warm-up activities helps to make the penile tissues more malleable and sensitive to the Jelqing procedure. If you want to add effective warm-up activities into your regimen, here are some examples:

- Hot Towel Wrap: To start, soak a fresh towel in hot water that isn't boiling. After wringing out any extra water, wrap the warm cloth around your penis for five to ten minutes.

The heat facilitates blood vessel dilatation and penile tissue relaxation.

- Gentle Massage: After the genital area has been wrapped in a heated cloth, give it a little massage. Circular movements can be used to increase blood flow. This massage encourages relaxation in addition to improving blood circulation.

- Light Stretching: To further prepare the tissues, engage in mild stretching activities. Take little, gentle movements with the penis, holding each stretch for a few seconds. This enhances adaptability and preparation for Jelqing.

- Exercises for Kegels: Include Kegel exercises in your warm-up regimen. The pelvic floor muscles are contracted and relaxed during these workouts. Kegel exercises can improve the efficacy of Jelqing and aid in overall pelvic health.

By including these warm-up exercises into your routine, you will be able to create an ideal environment for jelqing, which will prepare the penile tissues for the regulated and rhythmic motions that are characteristic of this exercise. Following the completion of the warm-up, you will be able to go on to the detailed tutorial of making jelqing.

Step-by-Step Guide to Jelqing

Jelqing is performed by moving the penis in a semi-erect position while making controlled, repetitive strokes along its length. The objective is to stimulate blood flow and maybe bring about improvements in penile girth as well as general sexual function. The following is a detailed guide to the Jelqing process:

Step 1: Warm-Up (Reiteration):

Emphasize the significance of the warm-up activities that were covered earlier in the conversation. The preparation of the penile tissues and the improvement of blood circulation are both essential components of this early phase.

Step 2: Partial Erection:

To get a partial erection, which is normally between fifty and seventy percent. This guarantees that the penis is flexible enough to do the activity, but it also prevents it from being completely erect, which carries with it the potential for harm.

Step 3: Lubrication:

Use a substantial amount of lubricant that is either water-based or silicone-based and apply it on the penis. It is vital to use lubrication throughout the jelqing procedure to lessen the danger of discomfort and minimize the amount of friction that occurs.

Step 4: OK Grip:

By encircling the base of the slightly erect penis with your thumb and fingers, you may create a "OK" hold. Make sure that the grip is solid, but not too tight so that you do not experience any pain.

Step 5: Base to Glans Stroking:

When you have the OK grasp in place, move your hand in a calm and controlled manner from the base of the penis to the glans (tip) of the penis. Approximately two to three seconds should be sufficient to finish the stroke perfectly.

Step 6: Alternate Hands:

Once you have finished a stroke with one hand, you should let go of the grip and do the stroke with the other hand. A constant beat should be maintained throughout the whole workout, and you should continue to alternate your hands.

Step 7: Controlled Pressure:

For every stroke, apply a controlled amount of pressure. The idea is to provide enough pressure so that blood travels the whole length of the penis, without using excessive force. Try different pressure settings to see what is most comfortable and productive for you.

Step 8: Repeat and Maintain Consistency:

For a predetermined amount of time—typically 10 to 15 minutes for beginners—repeat the stroking action. Aim for regular sessions rather than infrequent, intensive workouts since consistency is crucial.

Step 9: Cool Down:

Complete a mild cool-down after the Jelqing session. To assist relax the tissues, this may entail applying a cool—not cold—compress to the vaginal region.

It is of the utmost importance to stress that Jelqing should not result in any suffering or discomfort. If you suffer any severe pain or chronic discomfort, you should instantly cease the activity and either reevaluate your method or seek the advice of a healthcare industry specialist.

Finding Your Comfort Zone

To have a happy and productive time in Jelqing, it is vital to choose places where you feel comfortable. Every single person is one of a kind, and methods that are successful for one person might not be appropriate for another. Consider the following important factors to assist you in locating your zone of comfort:

- Start Gradually: If you're not familiar with Jelqing, begin with less intense and shorter sessions. As your body adjusts, progressively increase the duration and pressure. Heading into too-intense workouts might cause pain or harm.

- Pay attention to your body: During and after Jelqing, pay special attention to how your body feels. If you feel any pain, discomfort, or strange feelings, stop doing the exercise. When done properly, jelqing shouldn't be harmful.

- Try Different Techniques: Individual tastes may need adjusting jelqing techniques. To determine what is most comfortable and productive for you, play about with the pace, pressure, and grip.

- Track Your Progress: Keep a record of your advancements throughout time. While physical changes might not be apparent right away, general sexual health gains like increased blood flow and greater erection quality can be felt sooner.

- Take Individual Variables Into Account: Your body's reaction to Jelqing can be influenced by variables including age, general health, and pre-existing medical issues. When figuring out your comfort zone and creating attainable objectives, keep these things in mind.

- Avoid comparing your experiences or development to that of others. The experience of Jelqing varies from person to person and the outcomes might also differ.

Pay attention to your comfort, development, and welfare.

- Incorporate Variety: Jelqing is adaptable to your tastes. To keep the program comfortable and interesting, try varying the frequency of exercises, the length of sessions, or the method.

Being conscious, having patience, and being prepared to adjust are all necessary qualities for the process of finding your comfort zone, which is a continuous process. By making your health and comfort a top priority, you may create a Jelqing practice that is both positive and sustainable, and that is in line with the sexual wellness goals you want for yourself.

ADVANCED JELQING TECHNIQUES

The exploration of more complex techniques becomes a natural step for individuals as they go on their Jelqing journey. This is done to further boost the effectiveness of this activity. We are going to delve into advanced Jelqing techniques in this comprehensive guide. Some of the techniques that we will cover include incorporating Kegel exercises for a holistic approach, introducing variations for progression, and addressing common challenges that individuals may face while practicing advanced Jelqing.

Introducing Variations for Progress

It is essential to incorporate variation into every training plan, and Jelqing is not an exception to this rule. Not only does the introduction of variants keep the practice interesting, but it also tackles different elements of penile health. A few advanced Jelqing versions are listed below for your consideration:

1. Dry Jelqing: Although lubrication is used in standard Jelqing, some people choose the dry Jelqing technique. For many who find lubrication uncomfortable or messy, dry jelqing may be their favorite method because of its unique feeling.

2. V-Jelqs: These exercises entail applying pressure to the sides of the penis with two fingers arranged in a V shape. This version offers an alternative method of stimulation by focusing on the lateral parts of the erectile tissues.

3. Helicopter Jelqs: The strokes of a helicopter jelq include a circular action. Rotate the grip just before the following stroke after finishing a standard Jelqing stroke. This variant gives the workout more movement.

4. Overhand Jelqs: The overhand Jelq has an overhand grip in place of the conventional OK grip. This version may give a distinct stretching feeling and target various parts of the penis.

5. Uli#3 Squeezes: Uli#3 is a sophisticated squeezing method in which one hand is used to grab the penis' base and the other to grip the mid-shaft. This may result in increased pressure and engorgement since it produces a "double clamp" effect.

6. Orange Jelqs: To do an Orange Jelq, you must hold an orange with your thumb and fingers. This version can be useful for applying pressure to particular penile parts and modifying it as necessary.

Wherever incorporating sophisticated variants into your practice, it is essential to proceed with caution and gradually introduce them when possible. Pay special attention to how your body reacts, and if you feel any discomfort or adverse consequences, you should think about going back to the fundamentals before attempting more advanced methods again.

Incorporating Kegel Exercises

Incorporating Kegel exercises into your regimen, in conjunction with more advanced Jelqing methods, can help contribute to a more holistic approach to male sexual health. The Kegel exercises focus on the muscles of the pelvic floor, which are extremely important for sexual function as well as overall health and wellness. The following is an example of how to incorporate advanced Jelqing with Kegel exercises:

- Recognizing the Pelvic Floor Muscles: Recognizing the pelvic floor muscles is a prerequisite for doing Kegel exercises. These are the muscles you utilize to halt midstream urine flow or to stop gas from escaping.

- Isometric Contractions: Engage in pelvic floor muscular contractions. For a count of five, contract and hold the muscles, then release them. As you gain strength, progressively increase the number of repetitions from the beginning.

- Include Kegel exercises in your Jelqing sessions: As you do your strokes, contract and release your pelvic floor muscles in sync with them. This raises the genital muscles' total level of activation.

- Kegel exercises should be progressed gradually, much as Jelqing. Gradually increase the length of contractions and the amount of reps. To reap the rewards, you must be consistent.

- Combine with Edging: You might want to try combining Kegels with edging, which is a technique where you push yourself to the verge of an orgasm and then stop. The control over ejaculatory reflexes can be improved by this combination.

- Pay attention to your body: Observe the response of your pelvic floor muscles. Reduce the force of the contractions and seek medical advice if necessary if you feel any pain or discomfort.

You may strengthen your pelvic floor and perhaps enhance sexual performance and genital health by including Kegel exercises in your advanced Jelqing program.

Addressing Common Challenges

Individuals who are making progress with advanced Jelqing techniques may come into problems that demand them to pay attention and make adjustments during their journey. Taking preemptive measures to address these difficulties will guarantee that the experience is both pleasurable and safe. The following is a list of frequent difficulties that are related to advanced Jelqing, as well as techniques to defeat them:

- **Discomfort or Pain:**

Challenge: When attempting advanced versions, some people may feel pain or discomfort during or after Jelqing sessions.

Solution: Review your grip, pressure, and technique. Make sure you're not using too much force. Consider going back to the fundamental Jelqing techniques and introducing the advanced versions one at a time if discomfort continues.

- **Redness or Irritation:**

Challenge: Penile skin redness or irritation is possible, particularly after vigorous or protracted Jelqing.

Solution: Make sure you lubricate properly, hold the object gently, and keep an eye on how long your sessions last. Take a pause and let the skin recover if the irritation doesn't go away. To calm the skin, think about applying a hypoallergenic moisturizer.

- **Lack of Progress:**

Challenge: If they don't observe the anticipated improvements in terms of size or sexual function, some people might become disappointed.

Solution: Recall that every person will have different outcomes. Review your method, consistency, and strategy as a whole. Think about complementing workouts, leading a healthy lifestyle, and emphasizing the wider advantages of better sexual health.

- **Overtraining:**

Challenge: Excessive frequency and intensity of Jelqing, or overtraining, can result in discomfort, exhaustion, and other adverse consequences.

Solution: After each workout, give yourself enough time to relax and recuperate. When it comes to quality, quantity is secondary. Lower your session frequency and intensity if you exhibit overtraining symptoms, such as chronic fatigue or discomfort.

- **Emotional Stress:**

Challenge: Exercises for male enhancement might occasionally cause emotional strain or worry related to performance.

Solution: Maintain a cheerful outlook and reasonable expectations. Prioritize the process of achieving sexual well-being and self-improvement over focusing only on physical appearances. Should emotional strain continue, you might want to think about getting help from a mental health specialist.

People may confidently and adaptably manage the intricacies of advanced Jelqing procedures by overcoming these typical problems. The secret is to approach the exercise with awareness, a dedication to safety, and an openness to modify according to personal responses and requirements. People may confidently and adaptably manage the intricacies of advanced Jelqing procedures by overcoming these typical problems. The secret is to approach the exercise with awareness, a dedication to safety, and an openness to modify according to personal responses and requirements.

CREATING A JELQING ROUTINE

To go on a trip to Jelqing, it is necessary to build a routine that is both planned and durable. This is because the exercises themselves are only one component of the journey. In this extensive guide, we will discuss the essential components that are necessary for developing an efficient Jelqing routine. These components include the significance of maintaining a regular schedule, ensuring that workouts are balanced with sufficient rest, and monitoring progress in order to boost motivation and make necessary adjustments.

Establishing a Consistent Schedule

When it comes to completing a workout regimen, consistency is the most important factor, and Jelqing is no exception. This helps to integrate Jelqing into your everyday routine, which is necessary to make it a sustainable habit. Establishing a consistent timetable is crucial. Creating a Jelqing schedule that is constant may be done as follows:

- Establish Reasonable Goals: To start, decide on reasonable objectives for your Jelqing adventure. Whether your objective is to increase girth, improve sexual function, or support general genital health, having specific goals can help you stay on track.

- Pick a Convenient Time: Decide on a time of day that works well for your schedule. Consistency is crucial, regardless of the time of day—morning, evening, or any other time that works for your lifestyle. Include Jelqing in your regular self-care regimen.

- Make Frequent Sessions a Priority: Try to meet regularly for Jelqing sessions every day of the week. Although the number of sessions might vary depending on personal preferences, it's standard practice to begin with two to three per week and increase as your body adjusts.

- Include Jelqing in Your Daily Routine: Include Jelqing in all facets of your everyday activities. Whether you do it as part of your evening relaxation, during your workout, or right before or after the shower, finding a natural fit increases the probability of consistency.

- Employ Reminders: To help you remember to Jelqing, set alarms or reminders. Routine cues are typically beneficial to consistency, and reminders can help make Jelqing a daily habit.

- Adapt to Your Lifestyle: Realize that changes are inevitable in life and that your regimen may need to be modified. To ensure that

Jelqing continues to be a practical and fun activity, be adaptable and flexible with changes in your schedule.

To provide the groundwork for long-term success with Jelqing, you must first develop a regimen that is followed consistently. At this point, let's discuss the significance of ensuring that Jelq sessions are balanced with sufficient recuperation.

Balancing Jelq Workouts with Rest

While regularity is essential, finding a balance between Jelq exercises and enough recovery is just as critical. Excessive training may result in undesirable consequences, weariness, and reduced efficacy. To attain a harmonious balance, follow these steps:

- Put Quality Above Quantity: Place more emphasis on the caliber of your Jelqing sessions than the number of them. A regulated, well-executed workout yields greater benefits than a hurried or excessively strenuous one. Be mindful of your comfort and technique.

- Include Rest Days: Include rest days in your schedule to give your vaginal tissues time to heal. It makes sense for novices to begin with two to three sessions a week and work their way up from there. It's essential to take rest days to avoid overtraining.

- Pay Attention to Your Body: Keep a close eye on how Jelqing affects your body. If you continue to feel tired, sore, or exhibiting symptoms of overtraining, you might think about scheduling more rest days. A key part of muscle and tissue adaptation is rest.

- Change Intensity: If you use advanced Jelqing techniques, you might want to think about changing how intense your sessions are. You may, for instance, have a more strenuous session one day and a kinder one the next. This variant may aid in avoiding overdoing it.

- Recovery Methods: On days when you take a break, use recovery methods like warm compresses or light massages. These exercises help improve vaginal health generally and blood circulation.

- Hydrate and Sustain Nutrition: Eating a well-balanced diet and being properly hydrated is important for healing. Make sure you drink plenty of water and think about including foods high in vitamins and antioxidants that promote tissue health.

- Speak with Professionals: See a licensed fitness specialist or a healthcare provider if you are experiencing chronic pain or overtraining symptoms. They can offer advice on how to modify your regimen to better meet your unique requirements.

It is essential to strike a balance between participating in Jelq exercises and taking rest to maximize the advantages of this exercise and avoid any potential adverse effects. Now that we have that out of the way, let's discuss the significance of tracking your progress as a tool that is both instructive and motivating.

Tracking Your Progress

A helpful tool for motivation, correction, and a realistic assessment of the effectiveness of your Jelqing regimen is tracking your progress. This may be accomplished by keeping track of your progress. When it comes to efficiently implementing progress monitoring, this is how:

- Establish Baseline Measurements: Measure important factors including length, girth, and sexual function before beginning your Jelqing regimen. This gives future comparisons a point of reference.

- Use a Notebook or App: To record your sessions, either keep a Jelqing journal or utilize a specialized app. Provide information on the length of each session, any modifications or different approaches utilized, and any thoughts or emotions you had before and after the exercise.

- Regularly Reassess Your Objectives: Review your objectives from time to time and modify them in light of your advancement. This may be looking back at your original measurements, analyzing how your sexual function has changed, or thinking about any other advantages you've observed.

- Photographic Progress: To visually record changes, think about capturing pictures regularly. To ensure reliable comparisons, maintain constant lighting and angles. Beyond numerical metrics, photos may offer a tactile depiction of development.

- Recognize that it can take some time for changes to become apparent. Even little advancements are nevertheless advancements. You may strengthen a positive outlook and your dedication to your Jelqing program by keeping note of minor advancements.

- Celebrate Your Progress: Honor your progress made thus far. Celebrate and appreciate your accomplishments, whether they are meeting a certain measurement target, improving your sexual function, or just sticking to a regular schedule.

- Seek Professional Assistance: You should think about getting professional guidance if you have particular objectives or worries. A medical practitioner or a trained fitness specialist may give advice, modify your program, and assist you in setting reasonable goals.

- Changes Based on Feedback: Modify your routine with knowledge gained from the feedback you received from your progress monitoring. Try trying other strategies if particular methods or modifications aren't producing the expected outcomes.

You may make your Jelqing practice more dynamic and adaptable by keeping track of your advancement regularly. The knowledge gathered from tracking helps you make more educated decisions, stay motivated, and comprehend how Jelqing affects your unique experience with male sexual health.

COMPLEMENTARY EXERCISES AND PRACTICES

In addition to Jelqing, including complementing workouts and practices into your regimen can also aid in the general health of your male sexual organs. This all-encompassing book will provide you with information on stretching exercises that will improve your flexibility and blood flow, the influence that cardiovascular health has on sexual well-being, and nutritional assistance that will help you maximize your journey toward self-improvement.

Stretching Exercises

Stretching activities are essential for preserving blood flow, increasing general physical health, and preserving flexibility. Adding focused stretches to your exercise regimen can enhance the benefits of Jelqing. Consider the following particular stretching exercises:

- Stretches for the Pelvic Region: Pay particular attention to these stretches. Examples include butterfly stretches, which include sitting with your feet flat on the floor and gently pressing your knees toward the floor, and pelvic tilts, which involve lying on your back, contracting your abdominal muscles, and tilting your pelvis upward.

- Hamstring stretches: The general health of the pelvis depends on the hamstrings' flexibility. Stretch your hamstrings while seated or standing to increase the suppleness of your rear thighs.

- Hip Flexor Stretches: Improving pelvic mobility can be achieved by stretching the hip flexors. Targeting the hip flexors may be accomplished with both forward and backward lunges. Take care of your form to prevent strain.

- Lower Back Stretches: You may release tension in the lumbar area by doing gentle lower back stretches like the yoga pose known as the cat-cow stretch. Aim for fluid, deliberate motions.

- Whole-Body Stretching Program: Take into account adding a weekly full-body stretching routine to your agenda. Static stretches following a workout or Jelqing session and dynamic stretches before activity might be included in this.

- Pilates or yoga: Attending Pilates or yoga courses can offer systematic stretching routines that address various muscle groups. In addition to emphasizing breath control and awareness, these techniques improve the mind-body connection.

By including stretching exercises in your routine, you may improve your flexibility, lessen the stress in your muscles, and make a contribution to the general health of the pelvic area. Having said that, let's investigate the influence that cardiovascular health has on sexual well-being here.

Cardiovascular Health and Its Impact

Sexual health is a critical component of overall well-being. To achieve and sustain erections, effective blood flow is ensured by a healthy cardiovascular system. Cardiovascular exercise promotes general cardiovascular fitness in addition to supporting sexual function. The following are some tips for adding cardiovascular activities to your routine:

- Workouts That Raise Your Heart Rate: Engage in aerobic exercises that raise your heart rate. Exercises like cycling, swimming, dancing, running, and brisk walking are great options. Try to get in at least 150 minutes a week of aerobic activity at a moderate level.

- Interval Training: Include interval training, which alternates between brief sprints of intense activity and rest intervals at a reduced intensity. When it comes to increasing cardiovascular fitness, this method can be especially successful.

- Circuit Training: This type of training includes short rest intervals between sets of exercises designed to target various muscle groups. This kind of exercise increases general fitness as well as cardiovascular health.

- Stay Active Throughout the Day: Aim to maintain an active lifestyle outside of focused training sessions. To avoid extended stretches, walks, or moderate exercise, take regular pauses from inactive activity.

- Speak with Healthcare Specialists: Seek advice from healthcare professionals before beginning a new fitness program, particularly if you already have medical concerns. Based on your unique health situation, they can offer advice on the best cardiovascular workouts.

Cardiovascular activities have a direct influence on sexual function and also enhance mood, energy, and general well-being. As you give cardiovascular health priority, think about how it enhances the advantages of stretching and Jelqing activities in your all-encompassing strategy.

Nutritional Support for Sexual Well-being

Maintaining general health, including sexual health, is greatly aided by proper nutrition. A diet high in nutrients and well-balanced can help to maintain hormonal balance, improve blood flow, and support healthy sexual performance. The following food recommendations will help you on your path to bettering yourself:

- Balanced Diet: Make sure your diet is well-rounded by consuming a range of fruits, vegetables, whole grains, lean meats, and healthy fats. Foods high in nutrients offer vital vitamins and minerals that assist sexual function and general health.

- Hydration: Staying well hydrated is essential for both sexual and overall health. Water maintains healthy physical functioning, promotes blood circulation, and aids in controlling body temperature. Make it a daily goal to drink enough water.

- Omega-3 Fatty Acids: Flaxseeds, chia seeds, walnuts, and fatty fish (such as salmon and mackerel) are good sources of omega-3 fatty acids, which are good for the heart. Blood flow is important for sexual function and can be positively impacted by including these sources in your diet.

- Foods High in Antioxidants: Antioxidants protect the body from oxidative stress and inflammation. Eat a range of foods high in antioxidants, such as almonds, citrus fruits, dark leafy greens, and berries.

- Foods High in Zinc: Zinc is a mineral that is important for the synthesis of testosterone and general sexual health. Include foods high in zinc in your diet, such as beef, oysters, pumpkin seeds, and legumes.

- Steer clear of Too Much Alcohol and Caffeine: While some people may find that moderate alcohol use is okay, too much alcohol might have a detrimental effect on one's ability to conceive. Similarly, a lot of caffeine can cause anxiety and interfere with sleep, which can harm one's general health.

- Moderate Sugar and Processed Meals: Consuming excessive amounts of sugar or processed foods might worsen cardiovascular health by inflaming the body. Reducing the consumption of these items promotes sexual and general health.

- Speak with a Nutritionist: For individualized nutritional advice, think about scheduling a consultation with a nutritionist or other healthcare provider. They can offer advice based on your unique objectives, food choices, and health situation.

By adopting a nutrient-dense and balanced diet, you provide your body with the essential components it needs to function optimally. Nutritional support, when combined with Jelqing, stretching exercises, and cardiovascular health, contributes to a holistic approach to male sexual well-being.

MAINTAINING SEXUAL HEALTH

To ensure sexual health, it is necessary to take a holistic strategy that includes frequent checkups, lifestyle considerations, and psychological well-being. This is because ensuring sexual health entails more than just certain exercises and activities. Within the scope of this all-encompassing guide, we will investigate the significance of routine checkups for sexual health, the lifestyle factors that have the potential to influence sexual function, and the psychological aspects that play a significant role in the maintenance of sexual life that is both healthy and emotionally satisfying.

Importance of Regular Check-ups

Regular examinations are essential for maintaining general health, and maintaining sexual health is no different. Regular medical check-ups facilitate the early identification and treatment of any problems, which supports a proactive approach to sexual health. The following are important factors for routine check-ups:

- STI screening: It's critical to get regular testing for sexually transmitted infections (STIs), particularly if you engage in sexual activity. The prevention of future transmission of STIs as well as individual health are enhanced by early identification and treatment of STIs.

- Hormonal Health Evaluation: Routine check-ups offer a chance for evaluation for those who are worried about their levels of testosterone or other hormones. Sexual function can be impacted by hormonal imbalances, which can be resolved to promote well-being.

- Assessment of Cardiovascular Health: Sexual function and cardiovascular health are intimately related. Frequent examinations, which include measurements of cholesterol and blood pressure, help prevent and treat cardiovascular diseases that may have an impact on sexual health.

- Prostate Health: As people age, routine evaluations of their prostate health become crucial for those who were given a male gender at birth. Sexual function may be impacted by prostate disorders such as prostate cancer or benign prostatic hyperplasia (BPH). The key is early detection and action.

- Talking About Sexual Issues: Routine examinations offer a private, secure setting for talking about any issues you may be having with your sex. Having open lines of communication with medical staff can result in the proper advice, recommendations, or interventions when they're needed.

- Assessment of Mental Health: Sexual health and mental health are closely related. Frequent check-ups provide a chance to talk about mental health issues like sadness or anxiety that may affect one's ability to conceive.

- Monitoring General Health: General health has an impact on sexual health. Frequent examinations enable medical practitioners to keep an eye on a variety of well-being metrics, guaranteeing that possible problems are found and dealt with completely.

- Age-Related Assessments: As people become older, several health-related issues come into focus. Frequent check-ups offer chances for examinations that are suitable for a person's age, addressing issues that can come up at various periods of life.

To preserve sexual health, it is important to see routine examinations as a proactive and empowered procedure. Collaboration on well-being is facilitated by open communication with healthcare providers, who may address prospective problems as well as preventative actions.

Lifestyle Factors Affecting Sexual Function

The way of life that a person leads has a big impact on their sexual health and function. A healthy lifestyle may have a favorable effect on several things, including hormone balance and cardiovascular health. Here are some lifestyle elements to think about:

- Physical Activity: Engaging in regular physical activity promotes general well-being, blood circulation, and cardiovascular health. Take part in enjoyable workouts that combine strength training and cardiovascular activities.

- Healthy Diet: A well-rounded, nutrient-rich diet promotes sexual and general health. Include a range of entire grains, fruits, vegetables, lean meats, and healthy fats in your diet.

- Sustaining a Healthy Weight: Reaching and keeping a healthy weight can have a good impact on cardiovascular health and hormonal balance. It is essential for general health. Seek advice from medical specialists for specific recommendations on weight control.

- Limiting Tobacco and Alcohol: Excessive tobacco and alcohol usage might impair one's ability to have sex. Reducing or giving up these behaviors can help you have better sexual health.

- **Sufficient Sleep:** Getting enough good sleep is crucial for maintaining general health, which includes hormone balance and mental clarity. Aim for seven to nine hours of good sleep every night.

- **Stress management:** Prolonged stress might impair a person's ability to mate. Include stress-reduction strategies in your daily routine, such as yoga, meditation, mindfulness, and other forms of relaxation.

- Hydration: Keeping enough water in the body is essential for maintaining good blood circulation, preventing dehydration-related problems that might affect sexual health, and maintaining general health.

- Safe Sex Practices: Maintaining sexual health and avoiding STIs require the use of safe sex practices. Always wear protection, and be transparent with your partners about your sexual health habits.

- Review of Medication: Certain drugs may affect a person's ability to conceive. Consult a healthcare provider about your drugs if you have any concerns so that you may look into possible changes or substitutes.

- Preventing Illegal Drug Use: Using illegal drugs can hurt one's sexual health. Steer clear of them to enhance both sexual and general well-being.

Individuals may make a proactive contribution to their sexual health and general well-being by adopting a healthy lifestyle and making good lifestyle choices. It is common for beneficial adjustments in one aspect of one's lifestyle to lead to improvements in other areas. Lifestyle decisions are interrelated.

Psychological Aspects of Sexual Health

The mind-body link is important for sexual health, and a comprehensive approach must address psychological issues. Maintaining a healthy and meaningful sexual life requires careful attention to relationship communication, stress management, and emotional well-being.

Relationship Communication: Honest and open communication between couples promotes closeness, understanding, and trust. Talking about limits, worries, and wants helps to create a healthy and fulfilling sexual encounter for both parties.

Handling Mental Health Issues: Anxiety and depression are two mental health issues that can affect a person's ability to have sex. It's critical to get expert assistance for mental health issues. Psychologists, counselors, and therapists are qualified to offer assistance and direction.

Body Image and Self-Esteem: Sexual confidence is influenced by body image and self-esteem. Develop a healthy body image and sense of self-worth by accepting who you are, taking care of yourself, and recognizing your abilities.

Managing Stress: Sexual problems may arise from long-term stress. Include stress-reduction strategies in your daily routine, such as mindfulness, deep breathing, or partaking in enjoyable and relaxing hobbies.

Examining Sexual Wellbeing Practices: Take into consideration techniques that improve general sexual wellness, such as practicing mindfulness during personal interactions, indulging in sensuous activities, or using sexual health education materials.

Educational Materials: Use credible educational resources to stay up to date on sexual health issues. Having a better understanding of anatomy, sexual response, and typical problems may help one approach sexuality with greater confidence and health.

Counseling or sex therapy: Seeking the advice of a sex therapist or counselor can offer customized help for individuals or couples dealing with particular issues. These experts focus on resolving sexual issues and enhancing sex happiness.

Developing Emotional Closeness: Emotional intimacy improves a couple's relationship. Take part in activities that foster emotional intimacy, such as sharing stories, spending time together, and having open dialogue.

Examining Fantasies and Wants: Promote candid discussions about fantasies and desires in the framework of a courteous and cooperative partnership. Investigating common interests can lead to a more satisfying sexual life.

Taking care of psychological components includes valuing and promoting emotional health, cultivating wholesome connections, and getting help when required. There is a strong link between the mind and body, and having good mental health has a big impact on sexual health.

SAFETY AND PRECAUTIONS

To guarantee safety and reduce potential hazards, engaging in male enhancement activities, such as Jelqing and similar procedures, calls for a deliberate and cautious approach. This thorough guide will cover topics such as knowing the possible hazards of these activities, knowing when to consult a specialist, and how crucial it is to maintain general health to support a safe and successful male enhancement journey.

Understanding Potential Risks

It's important to understand the hazards involved and take the appropriate safety measures before starting any male enhancement workout program. Even though these activities may benefit a lot of people, being aware of the hazards might help people make wise judgments and adopt safe behaviors. The following are important things to remember:

- Overexertion and Damage: Overexertion, which can result in injury, is one of the main hazards connected to male enhancement activities. Strains, bruises, or other injuries to the genital area may arise from using improper techniques, applying too much pressure, or not providing enough time for recuperation.

- Allergies and Skin Irritation: Using lubricants or other materials while exercising may cause allergic responses or skin irritation. Selecting lubricants that are hypoallergenic and safe for the body is crucial. If discomfort arises, stop using the product and look for suitable relief.

- Damage to Vascular Structures: Improper or aggressive methods may result in damage to the vessels. This danger highlights how crucial it is to apply regulated pressure, adhere to proper technique, and monitor any pain throughout the exercise.

- Peyronie's Disease: This ailment results in the formation of fibrous scar tissue inside the penis, which can cause discomfort and curvature during erections. While there isn't enough proof to draw a firm conclusion, using excessive power or incorrect techniques during male enhancement exercises may increase the risk of developing Peyronie's disease.

- Psychological Stress: Taking part in male enhancement activities can cause psychological stress, especially if people have excessive expectations or become excessively focused on reaching particular goals. You must approach these workouts with a good outlook and attainable objectives.

- Pre-existing Ailments: Before beginning male enhancement workouts, those with pre-existing medical conditions, such as blood clotting disorders, cardiovascular problems, or genital anomalies, should use caution and speak with healthcare specialists.

Precautions to Minimize Risks:

Gradual Progression: Begin with simple workouts and work your way up to more complex ones. Injury risk increases when one rushes into vigorous routines. Pay attention to your body and adjust the amount of intensity to suit your comfort zone.

Proper Warm-up: Before beginning any male enhancement workouts, make sure you warm up properly. Warming up the vaginal tissues with a warm compress or mild massage helps get them ready for the workouts.

Accurate Methodology: Acquire and adhere to accurate methods for every workout. Injuries may result from improper form or overuse of force. Make use of reliable sources, educational materials, or advice from knowledgeable people.

Use a premium, body-safe lubricant to minimize friction when performing activities. Steer clear of chemicals that might trigger allergic responses or irritation. If irritation develops, stop using it and get a new lubricant.

Regular Monitoring: Keep a tight eye on your body's reactions both during and after workouts. Keep an eye out for any indications of pain, discomfort, or strange changes. If the problems are ongoing, think about changing your routine or consulting a specialist.

Scheduled Rest and Recovery: Make sure you leave enough time in between sessions for rest and recuperation. Excessive training might make you tired and raise your chance of getting hurt. When it comes to male enhancement activities, quality matters more than quantity.

Speak with Healthcare Specialists: Before beginning any male enhancement regimen, speak with healthcare professionals if you have any pre-existing medical issues or are worried about any possible hazards. They can offer tailored guidance according to your particular health situation.

Through a careful approach to male enhancement activities, people may reduce hazards and put safety first at every stage of their journey. An additional component of a safe and responsible strategy is realizing the value of expert counsel and maintaining general health.

When to Seek Professional Advice

While doing male enhancement exercises can be a voyage of self-improvement, there are situations in which consulting a specialist is imperative. Medical specialists may offer individualized advice, handle certain issues, and make sure people start male enhancement workouts safely. In the following circumstances, consulting a professional advisor is advised:

Pre-existing Medical Illnesses: Before beginning male enhancement workouts, speak with a healthcare provider if you have any pre-existing medical conditions, such as blood clotting disorders, cardiovascular problems, or genital anomalies. They can evaluate any hazards and offer customized guidance.

Persistent Pain or Discomfort: Seek expert assistance if you encounter odd feelings, pain, or discomfort during or after male enhancement workouts. If your discomfort doesn't go away with rest or gets worse over time, you might need to get evaluated.

Signs of Vascular Problems: You should visit a healthcare provider right away if you have any changes in the color, warmth, or feeling of your genital area. Vascular issues need to be evaluated and treated very often.

Skin Irritation or Allergic Responses: See a medical expert if you suffer from skin irritation, redness, or allergic reactions associated with lubricants or chemicals used during exercise. They can handle any dermatological issues and provide appropriate substitutes.

Fears Regarding Peyronie's Disease: Seek professional assessment if you experience discomfort during erections, see changes in penile curvature, or have worries regarding the development of Peyronie's disease. Medical practitioners are qualified to evaluate symptoms, carry out required testing, and offer pertinent advice.

Effect on Sexual Function: Seek medical advice if engaging in male enhancement activities has a detrimental effect on sexual function or causes problems like erectile dysfunction, changes in desire, or problems ejaculating. It could be necessary to thoroughly evaluate these issues.

Mental Health Impact: You should think about consulting a mental health expert if doing male enhancement activities causes you to experience a lot of psychological stress, anxiety, or body image issues. They can offer methods for addressing psychological well-being as well as assistance.

General Health Assessments: Regular general health evaluations, which include visits with medical specialists, offer a chance to talk about male enhancement techniques and handle any new issues that may arise. A proactive and comprehensive approach to well-being is ensured by regular communication.

It's critical to discuss male enhancement procedures with medical specialists honestly and openly. This makes it possible for them to offer knowledgeable and encouraging advice that takes into account both the psychological and physical components of the journey.

Maintaining Overall Health

The safety and efficacy of male enhancement activities are mostly dependent on an individual's general health. Making overall well-being a priority reduces possible dangers and helps create a supportive environment for these workouts. Key elements of preserving general health are as follows:

- Regular Check-ups: To keep an eye on your general health, schedule routine check-ups with medical specialists. These evaluations offer a forum for talking about male enhancement techniques, addressing issues, and making sure that workout regimens complement each person's health situation.

- Cardiovascular Health: Given its strong connection to sexual function, cardiovascular health should be given priority. Exercise your heart regularly, eat a balanced diet, and get frequent medical checkups to check your cholesterol and blood pressure.

- Hormonal Balance: Sexual wellness depends on hormonal balance. For proper evaluations, people should speak with healthcare providers if they have concerns about their hormone levels, regardless of whether they are caused by male enhancement workouts or other circumstances.

- Mental and Emotional Well-Being: Promote mental and emotional well-being by practicing relaxation methods, stress reduction, and honest discussion about issues or objectives. Dealing with psychological issues helps one have a good outlook while on the improvement path.

- Adopt a healthy, well-balanced diet that promotes general well-being. Make sure to include a range of healthful grains, fruits, veggies, lean meats, and healthy fats. Energy levels and general well-being are positively correlated with adequate diet.

- Sufficient Hydration: Maintain a sufficient level of hydration, as it is essential for several body processes. Blood circulation, which is essential to sexual function, is one aspect of general health that water aids.

- Prioritize getting a good night's sleep to aid in both your physical and emotional healing. For reliable and rejuvenating sleep, aim for 7-9 hours of sleep each night and develop healthy sleeping habits.

- Frequent Physical Exercise: Take part in frequent physical activity that suits your tastes and health. Engaging in physical activity promotes mood, cardiovascular health, and general well-being.

- Safe Sexual Behaviors: In addition to engaging in male enhancement activities, maintain your sexual health and avoid STIs by engaging in safe sexual behavior. Communicate freely and consistently with your sexual partners when using protection.

An individual may lay the groundwork for a path toward male enhancement that is both safe and successful by ensuring that they maintain their entire health. This comprehensive approach guarantees that male enhancement workouts are incorporated into a lifestyle that places a priority on well-being and reduces the likelihood

of potential hazards.

SUCCESS STORIES AND TESTIMONIALS

When beginning a path toward male improvement, such as by participating in activities like Jelqing, it is common practice to look to the experiences of others for inspiration and encouragement. The sharing of success stories and testimonials offers those who are on a similar route the opportunity to get encouragement and motivation by providing insights into real-life travels. In this all-encompassing book, we will investigate the real-life experiences of persons who have participated in male enhancement activities, as well as the encouragement and inspiration that may be obtained from these anecdotes.

Real-life Experiences

Success stories and testimonials that reveal real-life experiences offer insight into the many paths people take while pursuing male enhancement. It's critical to approach these narratives with the knowledge that different people may respond differently from one another and that what works for one person may not necessarily work for another. The following are some recurring motifs seen in actual experiences:

Enhanced Confidence: A lot of people say that their attempts to improve their masculinity have given them more self-assurance. Beyond the obvious benefits of physical development, this confidence may have an impact on relationships, self-perception, and general well-being, among other areas of life.

Positive Modifications to Sexual Function: Some people report experiencing positive modifications to their sexual function, such as stronger erections, more endurance, or more enjoyment. Many times, a variety of factors—including the exercises themselves and the general emphasis on sexual health—are blamed for these changes.

Exercises aimed at improving one's masculine appearance may frequently lead to a greater sense of self-awareness and self-discovery.

This increased consciousness might lead to a better comprehension of individual preferences, limits, and general sexual wellness.

Commitment to a Healthier Lifestyle: Adopting a healthier lifestyle is a common theme in success tales. This entails engaging in regular exercise, eating a well-balanced diet, drinking plenty of water, and attending to other elements of general well-being.

Patience and Persistence: The importance of these traits is a recurring theme in success tales. Realistic outcomes frequently need steady work over an extended period. People who tell their success stories frequently stress how crucial it is to remain dedicated to the process.

Results Variability: It's important to understand that there might be a lot of variation in the results. While some people could see noticeable improvements, others might see less dramatic changes or might prefer to concentrate on the advantages to their general well-being over noticeable physical changes.

Emphasis on Safety: Conscientious people who talk about their experiences frequently stress how important it is to maintain caution and safety when performing male enhancement activities. This entails using the right methods, paying attention to one's body, and getting help from a professional when necessary.

Encouragement and Motivation

Those considering or already doing male enhancement activities may find inspiration and motivation from reading success stories and testimonies. These stories frequently offer wisdom, advice, and a feeling of unity that encourages an optimistic outlook. Here are several ways that motivation and encouragement may be found in success stories:

Motivation to Get Started: Individuals contemplating male enhancement workouts may find motivation from success tales. Finding evidence that others have effectively traveled comparable paths might serve as the impetus to set off on one's own.

Developing Reasonable Expectations: Learning from other people's experiences aids in the development of reasonable expectations. Success tales frequently emphasize the slow pace of development and the necessity of patience and persistent work to bring about significant improvements.

Overcoming Obstacles: A lot of success tales provide advice on how to get beyond obstacles and failures. When people encounter comparable problems on their development journey, it might be helpful to see how others overcame challenges.

Building a Supportive Community: One way to do this is via sharing success stories with others. A sense of camaraderie is fostered by people sharing their experiences and expressing thanks for the support and guidance they have gotten from others in the community.

Honoring Minor Victories: Success narratives commemorate not just significant adjustments but also minor victories and significant turning points. A positive and inspiring mentality is enhanced by acknowledging and appreciating small victories.

Offering Useful Advice: Success stories frequently include useful guidance and recommendations on methods, resources, and lifestyle modifications that have worked well. Those looking for practical ways to improve their efforts may find this material useful.

Emphasizing the Holistic Approach: Motivational success stories frequently draw attention to the need for a comprehensive strategy for male enhancement. This covers things like general health, mental wellness, and incorporating improvement techniques into a well-rounded way of living.

Encouraging Consistency: Learning from other people's experiences serves to emphasize the need for consistency. Seeing the life-changing results of those who have regularly participated in exercise may serve as a source of inspiration for continuing the enhancing regimen.

Emphasizing Individual Variation: Success tales highlight the idea that different people will respond differently to workouts for male enhancement. Embracing their different journeys and avoiding comparing one's advancement to others is facilitated by this acknowledgment.

It's critical to view success tales from a stance of balance, acknowledging the diversity of personal experiences. Although these stories are inspiring and motivating, a person's personal objectives, interests, and health concerns should be taken into account in addition to these stories.

FREQUENTLY ASKED QUESTIONS (FAQS)

There are a lot of issues and interests to consider when navigating the world of male enhancement workouts. We will explore commonly asked questions (FAQs) about male enhancement in this extensive book, covering typical concerns and offering knowledgeable responses and advice to empower people on their path. This book attempts to offer thorough information to assist people investigating the area of male enhancement, from comprehending the fundamentals to requesting clarification on safety and efficacy.

Common Queries Addressed

Q1: How does Jelqing operate, and what is it?

Answer: Jelqing is a physical stretching and massage technique intended to enlarge and enhance the penis's functionality. It entails positioning the penis in a semi-erect position and gradually massaging it rhythmically with a lubricant, ostensibly to encourage blood flow and tissue growth.

Q2: Are workouts for male enhancement safe?

Answer: Male enhancement exercises can be safe for a lot of people as long as they are done carefully and according to the right procedures.

Overexertion, damage, and skin irritation are among the possible concerns, though. It's essential to take safety precautions, begin with simple activities, and speak with medical specialists if you have any pre-existing health issues.

Q3: How long do male enhancement workouts take to show results?

Answer: Each person experiences effects at a different pace. While some people could see changes in a matter of weeks, others might need many months. The most important things are patience, good technique, and consistency. It's critical to have reasonable expectations and concentrate on the advantages for general well-being.

Q4: Can an exercise program for male enhancement permanently improve penis size?

Answer: Although some people claim to have temporarily increased in size before, during, and after exercise, there is disagreement on long-term size changes. Exercises for male enlargement may or may not be beneficial, and any apparent increase in size may depend on things like better tissue health and blood flow.

Q5: Are there any age limitations on exercising for male enhancement?

Answer: While not all age limits apply, prudence is suggested. While older people may exercise with an eye toward general health, younger people should concentrate on natural growth and development. It is advised to speak with medical specialists, particularly for people who already have health issues.

Q6: Is there a suggested fitness regimen for male enhancement?

Answer: A suggested regimen usually consists of warming up, working out, and giving yourself enough time to cool down. It is advisable to begin with simple workouts and work your way up gradually. There is no one-size-fits-all regimen, so people should customize their approach according to their level of comfort, their objectives, and their general health.

Q7: Do workouts for male enhancement promote sexual function?

Answer: Some people report increased stamina and erections, among other changes in sexual performance. By encouraging blood flow and tissue health, the workouts may improve general sexual health. Individual reactions differ, though, so it's best to consult a specialist if you have any specific sexual difficulties.

Q8: Are there other male enhancement options than Jelqing?

Answer: Absolutely, there are several other male enhancement exercises and methods available, such as kegel exercises, stretching exercises, and the usage of equipment like penile pumps. Every strategy has its supporters and drawbacks, so people should select strategies that suit their comfort zones and tastes.

Q9: Can there be negative consequences or injury from male enhancement exercises?

Answer: Injuries, skin irritation, or pain might result from improper practices, overexertion, or disregarding safety procedures. It's critical to use the right methods, pay attention to your body's cues, and get expert help if anything goes wrong.

Q10: *Should I see a doctor before beginning an exercise program for male enhancement?*

Answer: Absolutely, it is essential to speak with medical specialists, particularly for those who already have health issues. Experts may evaluate any hazards, give tailored recommendations, and provide direction on how to include male enhancement workouts in a comprehensive health regimen.

Expert Answers and Insights

Q11: What elements are included in the male enhancement exercises' efficacy?

Answer: Male enhancement exercise success is dependent on several elements, such as individual reaction, general health, correct technique, and consistency. Adopting a comprehensive strategy that takes into account lifestyle elements like mental and cardiovascular health may help provide favorable results.

Q12: Are there any particular safety measures that people should take?

Answer: Starting with simple workouts, implementing appropriate warm-up and cool-down routines, utilizing body-safe lubricants, and refraining from employing excessive or aggressive force are all examples of safety measures. Important safety precautions include keeping an eye out for any indications of pain and seeking advice from medical experts if necessary.

Q13: Do activities for male enlargement affect mental health?

Answer: Male enhancement activities can have both beneficial and bad psychological impacts. While improvements in self-esteem and confidence are typical, an overly fixation on reaching predetermined goals can cause stress.

It's critical to strike a balance between physical and mental health goals.

Q14: What part does general health play in the effectiveness of workouts for male enhancement?

Answer: Overall health, including cardiovascular health, hormonal balance, and mental well-being, significantly influences the success of male enhancement exercises. A balanced lifestyle, incorporating healthy habits and regular check-ups, supports the body's ability to respond positively to enhancement efforts.

Q15: Do activities for male enlargement affect sexual relationships?

Answer: Positive alterations in confidence and sexual function may have a beneficial effect on romantic relationships. It is recommended to have open discussions regarding enhancing procedures and goals with partners. Prioritizing mutual consent, understanding, and emotional connection is crucial in any kind of partnership.

Q16: Are there any particular workouts designed to treat erectile dysfunction?

Answer: Even while certain workouts for male enhancement may promote blood flow and erectile function, treating erectile dysfunction frequently necessitates a multifaceted strategy.

For those with erectile dysfunction issues, seeking advice from medical experts and thinking about medical procedures or therapies may be essential.

Q17: How can people maintain their motivation when they are making improvements?

Answer: Setting realistic goals is essential to staying motivated. The effectiveness of male enhancement techniques is significantly influenced by overall health, which includes cardiovascular health, mental clarity, and hormonal balance. A healthy lifestyle that incorporates regular check-ups and positive habits increases the body's ability to respond positively to attempts at rehabilitation. Moreover, acknowledging modest victories, looking for professional or community assistance, and emphasizing the advantages to one's general well-being. Sustaining motivation may be achieved by keeping an optimistic outlook, appreciating accomplishments, and modifying routines as necessary.

Q18: Are those with pre-existing medical conditions given special consideration?

Answer: Before beginning male enhancement workouts, those with pre-existing medical concerns should use caution and speak with healthcare providers. Experts may offer customized guidance, evaluate any hazards, and suggest adjustments depending on each person's unique health situation.

Q19: Can the efficacy of male enhancement workouts be affected by lifestyle factors?

Answer: Yes, a healthy diet, regular exercise, stress reduction, and enough sleep all have a beneficial effect on how effective male enhancement activities are. An all-encompassing strategy that attends to general health fosters an atmosphere that is conducive to improvement initiatives.

CONCLUSION

Starting a male enhancement journey requires a thorough awareness of the complexities involved, especially when doing activities like Jelqing. This book has made an effort to offer a comprehensive examination of some topics, from the fundamentals of Jelqing to handling safety issues, sharing success stories, and answering frequently asked questions.

The foundation for understanding male anatomy is laid by knowledge of the anatomy of the penis, the processes underlying blood flow and erection, and the significance of circulation for sexual health. Setting reasonable expectations, addressing common misconceptions, and taking safety precautions are all important aspects of getting started with Jelqing. Warm-ups, step-by-step instructions, and identifying one's comfort zone are key components of the improvement process, which is centered around basic and advanced Jelqing methods combined with a structured regimen.

Additionally, this book goes beyond Jelqing, including supplementary activities and routines that support whole sexual health. It has been investigated that stretching exercises, heart health, and nutritional assistance are essential elements of a comprehensive strategy. Furthermore, the necessity of preserving sexual health extends beyond physical activity, exploring the role of routine examinations as well as addressing psychological and lifestyle variables.

The careful consideration of safety and preventative measures highlights the appropriate pursuit of masculine improvement. Comprehending any hazards, obtaining expert guidance when required, and preserving general well-being emphasize the dedication to well-being during the enhancement process. Testimonials and success stories highlight the uniqueness of the upgrading process while providing inspiration and support by giving real-life insights into the range of experiences people have.

Frequently asked questions have been carefully answered, offering explanations for frequently asked issues and professional advice to help people along their journey. This book tries to provide people with the information and understanding necessary to appropriately navigate the world of male enhancement, covering everything from the nuances of Jelqing to more general concerns about sexual health.

To sum up, there are several facets to male enhancement, including psychological, emotional, and physical components. Through the consolidation of knowledge on anatomy, procedures, safety, and success stories, this book seeks to enable people to take charge of their improvement path with self-assurance, accountability, and dedication to their overall well-being. We believe that this thorough investigation will be a useful tool for promoting an informed and proactive approach to male enhancement.